BRAND NEW
TOXIC SUPERFOODS

A Pocket Guide on How High Oxalate Foods Can Affect Your Health

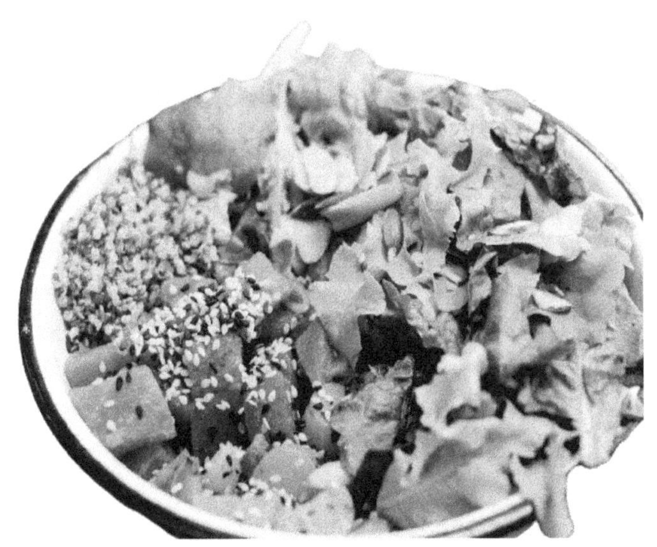

Dr. Ashley Voorhees

Contents

INTRODUCTION

Superfoods are ordinarily elevated as the key to ideal well-being and life, promising to improve energy, reinforce invulnerability, and even forestall affliction. Nonetheless, many individuals are unaware that some of these purported superfoods have a characteristic poison called oxalate that might be inconvenient to their well-being.

In this book, I will examine the secret dangers of oxalate and its effect on your well-being.

Oxalate is a molecule that is found in a lot of well-known superfoods, like spinach, kale, almonds, and products made from soy. While these food varieties are typically thought to be gainful, they may likewise be high in oxalate, related to various medical problems, including kidney stones, immune system issues, and even mind irregularities.

As of late, the fame of superfoods has expanded, with many individuals liking plant-based diets to better their well-being. In any case, the dangers of oxalate have generally been dismissed, with numerous well-being fans unconsciously consuming high levels of this poison consistently.

This book offers a complete manual for figuring out oxalate and its effect on your well-being. I will examine the science supporting this synthetic, the food varieties that contain it, and the well-being perils that might come about because of much gulping. If you have been affected by this toxin, I will discuss practical methods for reducing your oxalate intake and restoring your health.

Through this book, I desire to teach perusers about the dangers of oxalate and empower them to settle on guided decisions about their eating regimens and well-being. By understanding the effect of superfoods on the body, perusers might endeavor to safeguard themselves from the secret dangers of oxalate and carry on with a better, more energetic life.

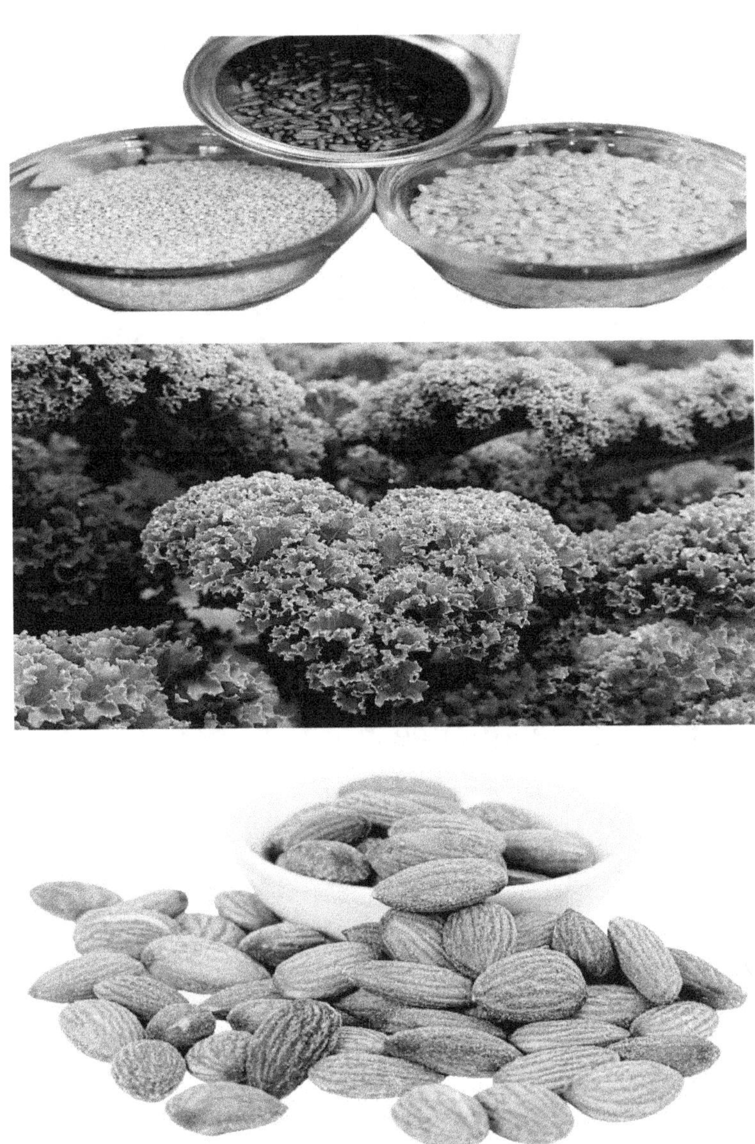

CHAPTER ONE

Superfoods are foods high in nutrients and are thought to have various health benefits. In recent years, their popularity has increased. Be that as it may, the maximum usage of these superfoods likewise has its dangers. One of the main issues that have become visible in many years is the presence of oxalates in these feasts, which might have extreme consequences for well-being.

What is Oxalate?

Oxalate is a characteristic, natural compound found in various plant sources. These foods are delicious because they usually have a lot of vitamins, minerals, and antioxidants. Nonetheless, oxalate is a poison that might harm the body when ingested at enormous levels. Oxalate is a translucent substance that creates sharp, needle-like designs, which might damage tissues and organs extensively.

For What Reason is it Unsafe to the Body?

Oxalate hinders the body since it is associated with minerals like calcium and produces insoluble calcium oxalate precious stones, which might accumulate in various body pieces, including the kidneys, urinary framework, and different organs. This gathering might cause many well-being troubles, including kidney stones, ongoing irritation, immune system infections, cerebrum irregularities like mental imbalance and Alzheimer's.

Oxalate Poisonousness Dangers

Oxalates are naturally occurring substances in various foods, including grains, nuts, fruits, and vegetables. They are framed when the body separates substances like L-ascorbic acid, which is additionally found in impressive sums in some superfoods. Consuming many oxalates can be harmful, but even small amounts can be detrimental.

At the point when oxalate levels in the body develop excessively high, they might solidify and cause kidney stones. This might cause extensive torment, nausea, and regurgitation. Kidney stones can cause kidney damage that will last a lifetime in severe cases. Oxalate harming may likewise prompt various well-being hardships, like joint touchiness, muscle shortcomings, and nerve harm.

Some superfoods high in oxalates incorporate spinach, kale, beets, almonds, cashews, and quinoa. When these feasts are regularly sound, individuals inclined to kidney stones or have a past filled with renal issues ought to be mindful while eating them.

Consuming these meals in moderation and balancing them with other healthy foods is essential to reduce the risk of oxalate poisoning. Moreover, drinking bunches of water could assist with flushing out extra oxalates from the body.

Realize that not all superfoods contain many oxalates, and many of them may provide significant health benefits without being toxic. Some low-oxalate superfoods incorporate blueberries, avocados, salmon, and chia seeds.

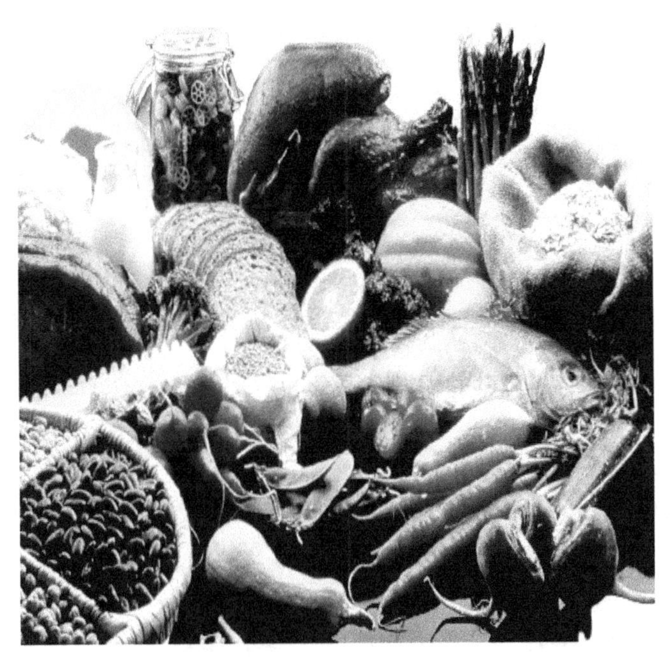

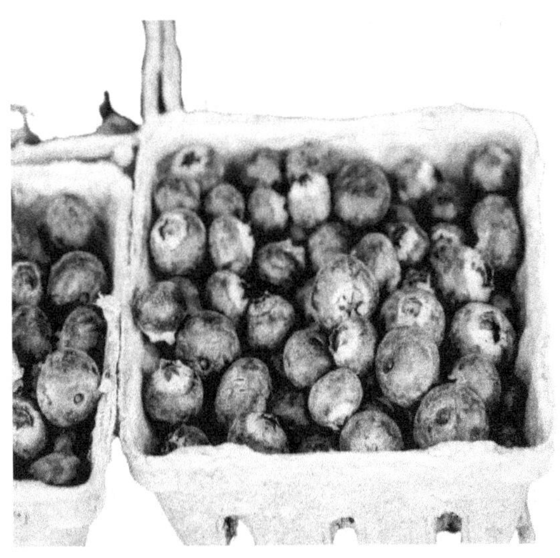

CHAPTER TWO

The Oxalate Science

Oxalate is a fundamental particle composed of two carboxylic corrosive gatherings (COOH) associated with a focal carbon molecule. Since carboxylic corrosive crowds are acidic, they might move a proton (H+) to a base. Oxalic corrosive has pKa upsides of 1.25 and 4.14, showing that it is a more grounded corrosive than acidic caustic (pKa = 4.76) and a more fragile corrosive than hydrochloric corrosive (pKa = - 7).

Oxalate might exist in a few structures in water, contingent upon the pH of the arrangement. At low pH, oxalate happens for the most part as totally protonated oxalic corrosive ($H_2C_2O_4$) and mono-protonated oxalate particle ($HC_2O_4^-$). When the pH rises, the oxalate particle ($C_2O_4^{2-}$) becomes the overwhelming species. By losing two protons at very high pH levels, oxalate might make the oxalate dianion ($C_2O_4^{2-}$).

Oxalate has a high proclivity for metal particles like calcium (Ca^{2+}) and iron (Fe^{3+}). The presence of two carboxylic corrosive gatherings, which might frame coordination bonds with metal particles, represents this partiality. The advancement of an oxalate-metal particle coordination complex might bring about the precipitation of insoluble salts like calcium oxalate.

Calcium oxalate precipitation is a common place peculiarity in natural frameworks. It is, for instance, the principal part of kidney stones, which might be created when the oxalate content in the pee is excessively high. A few factors, including heredity, sustenance, and specific ailments, could affect the development of calcium oxalate gems in the kidneys.

Oxalate likewise takes part in various metabolic responses in plants and creatures. In plants, oxalate is a calcium particle capacity particle. It might again go about as a chelating specialist, aiding the preparation and transport of metal particles inside the plant. Oxalate might be shaped due to digestion in well-evolved creatures, entirely in the liver. High oxalate levels in the blood might prompt the development of calcium oxalate gems in the kidneys, causing kidney harm and other well-being concerns.

The Stomach Related Cycle and Oxalate Assimilation.

The Stomach-related process is the perplexing component that our bodies utilize to separate the food we devour into more modest particles that might be retained and used for energy, improvement, and fixing. The cycle incorporates different organs and proteins cooperating to change food into a structure the body can utilize.

Food is bitten and joined with spit in the mouth, where the Stomach-related process begins. Spit incorporates catalysts that start to debase carbs. The feast goes through the throat and into the Stomach, where it is further separated by Stomach corrosive compounds.

The feast arrives at the small digestive system, where most digestion happens. The small digestive tract is fixed with villi, minuscule finger-like expansions that upgrade the surface region and are considered more noteworthy assimilation. As the dinner goes through the small digestive system, pancreatic compounds and liver bile keep separating into more modest particles.

At last, the excess supplements and water enter the circulation system and are conveyed all through the body. The side effects are removed from the body as dung.

Allow me now to talk about oxalate retention. Oxalate is available in different food sources, including spinach, rhubarb, and chocolate. While minuscule amounts of oxalate are not dangerous, exorbitant levels might cause kidney stones to create.

Oxalate is caught up in the small digestive system during processing. It could be consumed latently, which implies that it simply diffuses over the digestive coating, or effectively, meaning that specific carriers convey it across the covering.

Oxalate might be wiped out by the kidneys or held in tissues throughout the body once ingested. At the point when oxalate levels are high, it might respond with calcium to create calcium oxalate gems, which can then develop in the kidneys and cause kidney stones.

Generally speaking, assimilation is a significant part of our bodies' ability to extricate supplements and energy from food. While oxalate retention is a characteristic part of the interaction, it's substantial to restrict your utilization of high-oxalate feasts to forestall well-being concerns.

When we consume oxalate-containing feasts, the particle enters our gastrointestinal system and begins to be separated by chemicals in the Stomach and small digestive tract. Since these catalysts don't altogether dissolve oxalate, they might go through the stomach-related framework unblemished.

The microbes that abide in the digestive organ can use oxalate. Some of these microorganisms might change over oxalate into different substances the body can retain or oust in the stool. Since not every person's stomach greenery is similar, specific individuals might be less successful at utilizing oxalate than others.

When consumed by the body, oxalate might enter the course and be moved to various tissues. Oxalate might communicate with calcium in the flow and make insoluble precious stones, which can be stored in tissues and organs. As recently expressed, this might bring about a scope of medical problems.

Oxalate Digestion and Disposal in the Body.

Oxalate is generally processed in the liver and kidneys. In the liver, a catalyst named alanine-glyoxylate aminotransferase (AGT) separates oxalate into glyoxylate. Glyoxylate may then be divided into different synthetics or turned into oxalate.

The kidneys channel the central part of the oxalate that enters the course and kill it in the pee. A few factors influence the amount of oxalate discharged in pee, including how much oxalate is taken in the food, the body's age of oxalate, and the viability of the kidneys in separating and discharging oxalate.

People with appropriate renal capability can successfully channel and dispose of oxalate, holding it back from aggregating in the body. Nonetheless, in individuals with explicit ailments or hereditary varieties, oxalate might develop in the body and cause kidney stones or other medical issues.

The Accompanying Elements Might Raise the Gamble of Oxalate Development

- Utilization of oxalate-rich food sources incorporates spinach, rhubarb, beets, almonds, and chocolate.

- Clinical infections that obstruct sustenance ingestion, like provocative entrail sickness, celiac illness, or bariatric medical procedures.

- Essential hyperoxaluria and intestinal hyperoxaluria are hereditary changes that modify oxalate creation or digestion.

- Certain medications, like antitoxins and Stomach settling agents, could influence the stomach microbiota and improve oxalate retention.

People should adopt a fair eating regimen with humble amounts of oxalate-rich food sources and remain hydrated to diminish the gamble of oxalate collection and kidney stone turn of events. If an individual has an ailment or a hereditary change that influences oxalate digestion, they might require additional actions to control their oxalate levels, like prescription or dietary limitation.

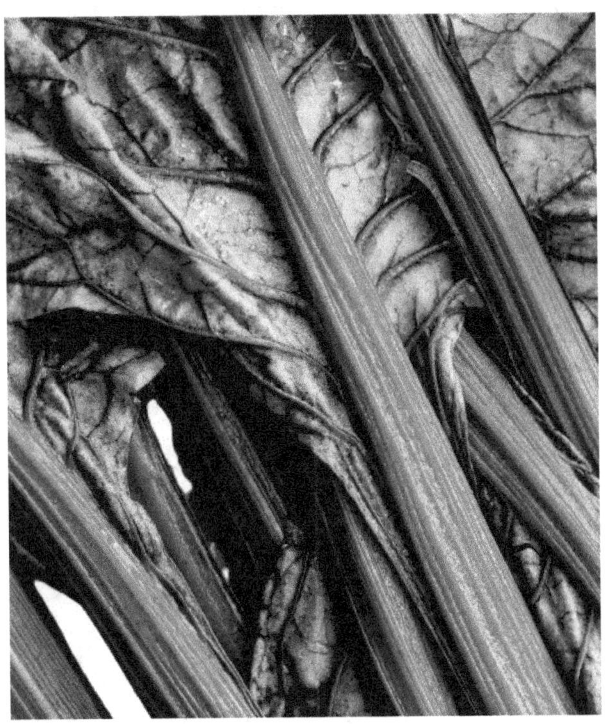

CHAPTER THREE

This chapter centers around the well-being effects of oxalate, especially its connection to kidney stones, immune system ailments, irritation, and neurological issues.

Kidney Stones: Causes, Side Effects, and Treatment Choices

Kidney stones are little, hard stores that fill in the kidneys and may cause extensive uneasiness when they travel through the urinary waterway. Oxalate is a critical part of most kidney stones, alongside calcium and minerals. At the point when oxalate levels are unreasonable, the additional oxalate might consolidate with calcium to make gems, which can eventually develop into kidney stones.

Side effects of kidney stones could include intense torment for the side or back, sickness and retching, fever, and chills. Treatment choices for kidney stones differ on the size and area of the rock, as well as the level of side effects. Choices might incorporate agony prescription, hydration, and, in uncommon conditions, medical procedures or other operations to eliminate the stone.

Forestalling kidney stones involves restricting the utilization of food sources rich in oxalate, like spinach, rhubarb, and beets. It's likewise urgent to drink enough water and have a sound eating routine and way of life.

Immune System Infections and Irritation

Immune system problems emerge when the invulnerable framework wrongly attacks the body's cells and tissues, prompting irritation and harm. Research shows that oxalate might contribute to immune system sicknesses by adding to irritation and oxidative damage.

Oxalate has been connected with numerous immune system ailments, including rheumatoid joint pain, lupus, and provocative gut illness. It's thought that an abundance of oxalate could upset the stomach verdure and increment gastrointestinal porousness, prompting irritation and safe framework initiation.

Lessening oxalate utilization and advancing stomach well-being through a reasonable eating routine and way of life might assist with diminishing irritation and further development of side effects of immune system sicknesses.

Oxalate and Neurological Problems

Neurological illnesses might be convoluted and intense to get a handle on. Specialists have looked at a likely connection between oxalate, mental imbalance, and different conditions. Oxalate is synthetic in numerous food sources, including mixed greens, almonds, and chocolate. It might likewise be created by the body and is removed in pee. At the point when oxalate develops in the body, it might add to a scope of unexpected issues, including neurological problems.

Chemical imbalance is a convoluted formative illness that hinders social communication, discourse, and conduct. It is a range condition, implying that the force and side effects might differ significantly from one individual to another. There is no known reason for mental imbalance, but hereditary qualities and ecological variables are likely to have an effect.

Late exploration has uncovered that over-the-top degrees of oxalate in the body might be related to the advancement of mental imbalance. Oxalate might influence the neurological framework by upsetting the balance of calcium and magnesium, two essential components for cerebrum capability. It might likewise advance aggravation, which has been connected with improving chemical imbalance.

One more problem related to oxalate is mitochondrial sickness. Mitochondria are the energy-delivering organelles in cells, and mitochondrial glitch has been connected with neurological disorders. High measures of oxalate might harm mitochondria, prompting energy creation issues and neurological side effects.

Other oxalate-related illnesses include persistent weariness, fibromyalgia, and peevish inside disorder. These issues are comparatively associated with mitochondrial brokenness and irritation, showing that oxalate might play a part in their turn of events.

One issue in analyzing the connection between oxalate and neurological diseases is that oxalate levels may be challenging to measure. The most reliable strategy is using a 24-hour pee test, but this is always beyond the realm of possibilities. Nonetheless, a few scientists are exploring novel ways of surveying oxalate levels in the body.

Treatment for high oxalate levels frequently incorporates dietary changes, like restricting the utilization of oxalate-rich food sources and expanding the admission of calcium and magnesium. Enhancements and medications may likewise be utilized to bring down oxalate levels. Further review is expected to find the ideal treatment methods for neurological issues associated with oxalate.

CHAPTER FOUR

This section tends to the oxalate content of superfoods, including salad greens, nuts, plant-based proteins, and foods grown from the ground.

Salad greens, like spinach and kale, are ordinarily hailed as superfoods inferable from their high nutrient substance. Be that as it may, these greens are likewise wealthy in oxalates. Spinach, in occurrence, has one of the most excellent oxalate groupings, everything being equal. Other mixed greens, such as Swiss chard and beet greens, also contain significant amounts of oxalates.

Spinach: Spinach is a famous verdant green vegetable with nutrients and minerals. Notwithstanding, it is additionally wealthy in oxalate, with 1 cup of cooked spinach having approximately 970 milligrams of oxalate.

Kale: Kale is one more rich green vegetable often advanced as a superfood inferable from its high nutrient substance. Notwithstanding, similar to spinach, it is additionally rich in oxalate, with 1 cup of cooked kale having approximately 1100 milligrams of oxalate.

Beet Greens: Beet greens are the verdant highest points of beets and are wealthy in oxalate. One cup of cooked beet greens contains around 910 milligrams of oxalate.

Swiss Chard: Swiss chard is a verdant green vegetable connected with beets and spinach. It is plentiful in various nutrients and minerals. However, it is likewise high in oxalate, with 1 cup of cooked Swiss chard having about 960 milligrams of oxalate.

Almonds: Almonds are a well-known nut regularly included in superfood records attributable to their highly nutritious substance. Be that as it may, they are additionally wealthy in oxalate, with 1 ounce of almonds having about 140 milligrams of oxalate.

Quinoa: Quinoa is a typical grain-like seed often viewed as a superfood inferable from its high protein content. In any case, it is additionally wealthy in oxalate, with 1 cup of cooked quinoa having approximately 280 milligrams of oxalate.

Soy merchandise: Soy items like tofu, tempeh, and soy milk are regularly highlighted in superfood records attributable to their high protein content and conceivable medical advantages. Notwithstanding, they are additionally wealthy in oxalate, with tofu conveying around 58 milligrams of oxalate for every 100 grams.

Nuts are one more sort of superfood that are rich in oxalates. Almonds and cashews are exceptionally high, albeit different nuts like pistachios, hazelnuts, and pecans additionally contain vast amounts of oxalate. Albeit nuts are a nutritious wellspring of protein and solid fats, people with a background marked by kidney stones ought to take them with some restraint.

Organic products and Vegetables that Contains oxalate

Leafy foods that contain oxalates incorporate berries, kiwi natural products, rhubarb, beets, and yams. Some of these food varieties, for example, berries and kiwi natural products, are high in different supplements and cell reinforcements, making them significant increments to a sound eating routine. Nonetheless, people in danger of kidney stones ought to take these things with some restraint.

In synopsis, oxalate is contained in a few superfoods, including verdant green vegetables, nuts, and seeds. While ingesting these food varieties with some restraint is typically respected as suitable for the vast majority, people with a background marked by renal infection or calcium oxalate kidney stones should talk with their medical care proficient about their oxalate utilization to guarantee they are not overeating.

CHAPTER FIVE

Instructions to Bring Down the Oxalate Diet to Stay Away from the Production of Kidney Stones

This chapter offers techniques for decreasing oxalate utilization, various nutrients to consider, and the job of enhancements and medication.

The first and best method for lowering your oxalate diet is to stay away from high-oxalate food sources. Instances of high-oxalate food sources include spinach, rhubarb, beets, okra, Swiss chard, peanuts, almonds, pecans, soy items, wheat grain, and buckwheat. By reducing the use of these things, you can extraordinarily reduce your oxalate consumption.

Cook Your Food: Preparing your food can assist with bringing down the oxalate level. Bubbling, warming, and baking are excellent approaches to reducing oxalate levels in food. For instance, cooking spinach briefly can decrease its oxalate level by up to half.

Drink Much Water: Drinking much water can assist with diminishing the amount of oxalate in the urine, reducing the risk of stone development. Mean to consume somewhere around 2–3 litres of water each day.

Elective Superfoods to Consider are:

Low-Oxalate Vegetables: Vegetables low in oxalate include kale, collard greens, broccoli, cabbage, cauliflower, and Brussels sprouts. These veggies are likewise high in calcium, which can assist with restricting oxalate in the stomach and blocking its assimilation.

Organic Products: Organic products low in oxalate include cherries, apricots, oranges, peaches, plums, and pears. These food varieties are likewise high in water content, which can assist with flushing out the kidneys.

Low-Fat Dairy: Low-fat dairy items, like milk, yoghurt, and cheddar, are great wellsprings of calcium and can assist with reducing oxalate in the stomach.

Notwithstanding, it's vital to make low-fat decisions and try not to eat much-saturated fat. The job of enhancements and drugs enhancements and medication can play a part in overseeing oxalate openness in more ways than one:

Physician-Recommended   Drugs: Certain doctor-prescribed medications can likewise assist with diminishing the chance of kidney stones by bringing down oxalate levels in the urine. For instance, potassium citrate can help make pee less acidic, reducing the development of calcium oxalate kidney stones. Moreover, the medication allopurinol can reduce uric acid in the body, which can assist with staying away from kidney stones.

Calcium Enhancements: Calcium enhancements can assist with restricting oxalate in the stomach and keeping it from assimilation. Be that as it may, it means a lot to take calcium tablets with dinner to work on their ingestion and to try not to take an excess of calcium.

Magnesium Enhancements: Magnesium can assist with staying away from the formation of calcium oxalate stones by forestalling the crystallization of calcium and oxalate in the pee.

Potassium Citrate: Potassium citrate can assist with working on the pH of the pee, making it less acidic and preventing the development of calcium oxalate stones.

Allopurinol: Allopurinol is a medication that can assist with bringing down the development of uric acid, which can prompt the action of kidney stones.

L-ascorbic Acid Pills: High doses of L-ascorbic acid pills can be converted to oxalate in the body, which can increase the risk of kidney stones. Subsequently, individuals in danger of kidney stones ought to decrease their L-ascorbic acid intake to something like 1,000 mg daily.

Probiotics: Some reviews show that particular kinds of probiotics might assist with bringing down oxalate retention in the stomach.

Notwithstanding, more review is required here to conclude which types are generally valuable and the amount to take.

Plant Pills: There are likewise a few plant pills that are elevated for their capacity to bring down the risk of kidney stones. Notwithstanding, the evidence backing their handiness is limited, and some might try to be hazardous in high amounts. Thus, individuals should constantly talk with a medical services supplier before taking any plant items.

Reducing your oxalate diet is a compelling method to avoid kidney stones. Systems for lessening oxalate utilization incorporate staying away from high-oxalate food sources, preparing your food, having much water, and taking restricted L-ascorbic acid pills. Elective superfoods to consider incorporate low-oxalate veggies, organic products, and low-fat foods.

CHAPTER SIX

"The Plant Conundrum" offers a manual for bringing down the adverse consequences of oxalates through food strategies and regular medicines. By adhering to these rules, individuals can develop their stomach well-being, support liver capability, decrease aggravation and oxidative pressure, and advance kidney well-being, all of which can assist with diminishing the adverse consequences of oxalates and work on broad well-being and prosperity.

Dietary Methodologies for Decreasing Irritation and Oxidative Pressure
Aggravation and oxidative pressure are two significant variables that improve constant

illnesses like coronary illness, diabetes, and disease. Luckily, there are a few food strategies that can assist with bringing down irritation and poisonous pressure in the body.

Eat an Eating Routine Wealthy in Cell Reinforcements: Cell reinforcements are substances that help kill free extremists, particles that can hurt cells and add to irritation and oxidative pressure. The best wellsprings of cancer prevention agents incorporate organic products, such as veggies, nuts, seeds, and entire grains. Food sources exceptionally high in cancer prevention agents include berries, new greens, yams, and flavors like ginger and cinnamon.

Increment Omega-3 Unsaturated Fat Admission: Omega-3 unsaturated fats are great fats tracked down in greasy fish, pecans, chia seeds, and flaxseeds. These fats assist with diminishing irritation and oxidative pressure in the body by bringing down the creation of supportive and provocative atoms called cytokines. Integrating more omega-3 unsaturated fats into your eating regimen can assist with bringing down irritation and safeguard against persistent sickness.

Stay Away from Refined Carbs: Refined carbs, like white bread, pasta, and sweet beverages, can cause a quick expansion in glucose levels, which can prompt irritation and oxidative pressure. Center around eating complex carbs like grains, veggies, and beans that give delayed energy and are less likely to cause aggravation.

Limit Immersed and Trans Fats: Soaked and trans fats are awful fats that can cause irritation and harmful pressure. They are often tracked down in handled and seared food varieties and in creature products like meat and cheddar. All things being equal, it centers around practicing good eating habits with fats like olive oil, avocado, nuts, and seeds.

Consolidate Aged Food Varieties: Matured food varieties like pickles, kimchi, and kefir are rich in supportive microbes that can assist with bringing down aggravation and oxidative pressure in the stomach. These accommodating microbes likewise support the safeguard framework and work on broad well-being.

Standard Solutions for Advancing Kidney Well-being

The kidneys are significant organs that assist with eliminating waste and additional liquid from the blood. Constant kidney infection is a typical sickness that can prompt kidney disappointment whenever left uncontrolled. Luckily, a few regular medicines can assist with supporting kidney well-being.

Remain Hydrated: Drinking much water can assist with flushing out poisons and preventing the development of kidney stones. You should drink no less than eight glasses of water a day; from there, the sky's the limit on the off chance that you are genuinely occupied or live in a hot climate.

Eat a Solid Eating Regimen: Eating a sound eating routine that is low in salt and includes well-handled food varieties can assist with safeguarding the kidneys from harm. Center around eating a lot of organic products, veggies, entire grains, and lean protein sources.

Work-out Routinely: Ordinary activity can assist with further developing kidney well-being and lowering the risk of kidney infection. Hold back nothing for 30 minutes of moderate-power practice most days of the week.

Utilize Home-grown Cures: Certain spices like dandelion, bother, and parsley can further develop kidney well-being by raising the pee stream and releasing aggravation in the kidneys. These leaves can be eaten as tea or taken as an enhancement.

Screen Circulatory Strain and Glucose: Hypertension and high glucose might add to kidney damage at any point. Observing your pulse and glucose levels daily can assist with staying away from kidney harm and advancing general kidney well-being.

In a rundown state, further developing kidney well-being and reducing irritation and oxidative pressure can be accomplished through food and lifestyle changes. Consolidating supplement thick food varieties, restricting unhealthy foods, and taking part in standard actual activity can assist with working on broad well-being and prosperity while bringing down the opportunity of constant diseases.

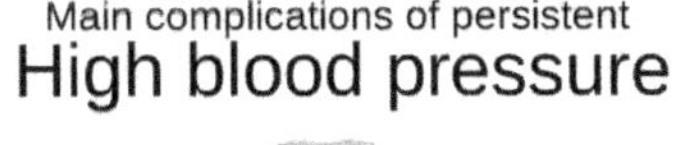

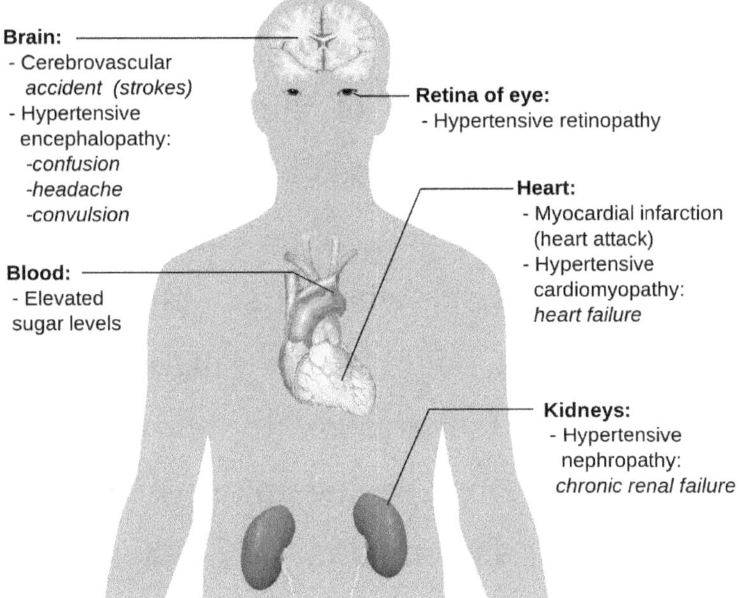

CHAPTER SEVEN

Self-Strengthening for Ideal Well-being

The primary variable is understanding the science fundamental to the supposed medical advantages of superfoods. While numerous superfoods have logical sponsorship for their cases, some might be overhyped past what the information upholds. You might make taught choices about which superfoods to add to your eating routine by keeping up to speed on the most recent examination and have some misgivings of well-being claims.

As well as being proficient in superfoods, it is essential to advocate for you and your well-being in the general public, where these food varieties are frequently promoted as "marvel fixes." It likewise involves taking a functioning part in your well-being, for example, teaming up with a trustworthy medical care professional and pursuing steady decisions with your convictions and desires.

At last, the way to the most extreme well-being is to move toward sustenance and health in a decent, all-encompassing way. Superfoods might be an incredible enhancement to a proper eating regimen. However, they are only one piece of the jigsaw. Getting satisfactory rest, controlling pressure, and remaining genuinely dynamic is fundamental to keeping up with social ties. You can engage yourself to carry on with your best life and get every one of the compensations by focusing on these parts of well-being and prosperity.

In this reality where superfoods are frequently promoted as "marvel fixes," how might you advocate for yourself and your well-being?

Supporting you and your well-being might be troublesome, especially in a general public with an overflow of well-being and nourishment information. Superfoods are frequently promoted as "supernatural occurrence fixes" for restoring any condition that might be dishonest and perilous. To advocate for yourself and your well-being, you should have glaring doubts about the data offered and go with instructed decisions given reliable sources.

Do Your Review: An exhaustive study is essential before endeavoring any new superfood or well-being supplement. Search for dependable sources, like logical investigations, to realize what the proof says regarding the conceivable well-being benefits and risks of a specific food or supplement. Abstain from putting together your choice just concerning advertising guarantees or recounted confirmation.

Talk to a Specialist: Before endeavoring any new well-being supplement or rolling out any improvements to your eating routine, it is generally wise to converse with a medical services master. A specialist or qualified dietitian can assist you with understanding the potential benefits and risks of bringing new food sources into your eating regimen and guaranteeing that they slow down no drugs you are taking.

Adopt a Fair Strategy: While superfoods may give specific well-being benefits, moving toward eating reasonably is basic. A different diet should contain organic products, vegetables, entire grains, lean meats, and solid fats rather than zeroing in on a few guaranteed "wonder" food sources centred around a decent and broadened diet.

Pay attention to Your Body: Everybody is unique, and what works for one individual may not work for another. Observe how your body responds to various dinners and substances. Talk with a medical care master if you have any horrendous responses or changes in your well-being.

Be Careful with Sham Cases: Tragically, numerous fake cases regarding the well-being benefits of superfoods and supplements exist. Any item that makes irrational or misrepresented guarantees regarding its potential benefits ought to be avoided. Recall that no body's diet or supplement can treat all illnesses or give each of the accessories your body requires.

Taking a Fair, All-encompassing Way to Deal with Nourishment and Health

A fair, all-encompassing way to deal with nourishment and health involves seeing well-being and prosperity comprehensively and recognizing the reliance on numerous components of our lives. This approach considers what we eat and how we work out, rest, manage pressure, and associate with others. Here are some vital components to recollect while chasing after a comprehensive way to deal with nourishment and health:

Eat a Supplement Thick Eating Regimen: A scope of complete food varieties is fundamental for obtaining the accessories our bodies need to work appropriately. Leafy foods, entire grains, lean meats, and solid fats are entirely suggested. Eat a rainbow of varieties to guarantee you get many supplements.

Observe Your Body: Our bodies are assorted and dynamic, and our dietary prerequisites could change depending on age, orientation, practice level, and well-being state. Focusing on how different feasts cause you to feel could assist you with pursuing more taught dietary decisions.

Move Your Body Consistently: Actual activity is helpful in general well-being and may assist with limiting the gamble of constant ailments. Find things you love and endeavour to incorporate development into your daily practice, whether it's strolling, yoga, strength preparation, or one more activity.

Rest should be focused on since it is essential for general well-being and prosperity. Go for long rest periods consistently and adhere to a standard rest timetable to help your body sink into an example.

Stress the Executives: Persistent pressure might adversely affect physical and psychological wellness. Stress-the-board practices like reflection, yoga, and other unwinding methods might help upgrade general prosperity.

Foster Social Ties: Social help is fundamental for physical and psychological wellness because people are social creatures. Make time to associate with loved ones, and search for excellent chances to reward your local area.

By incorporating these thoughts into your daily existence, you might take on a comprehensive way to deal with nourishment and well-being that advances ideal well-being and prosperity. Remember that minor adjustments amount to enormous benefits over the long run, and what turns out best for you requires some experimentation. You might lay out a sound way of life that meets your necessities and goals by being patient and tenacious.